MW01169430

IVERMECTIN

A comprehensive guide on how the medication could save millions of lives and put an end to the global pandemic

Dr Ronald L. Bell

Copyright © 2024 Dr Ronald L. Bell

All rights reserved. No part of this publication may be reproduced, distributed, or transmitted in any form or by any means, including photocopying, recording, or other electronic or mechanical methods, without the prior written permission of the publisher, except in the case of brief quotations embodied in critical reviews and certain other noncommercial uses permitted by copyright law.

Disclaimer

This book's content is meant to be used for informative purposes only; it is not intended to be a replacement for expert medical or veterinary advice. See a licensed healthcare provider or veterinarian before using Ivermectin or any other prescription. They can evaluate your unique needs, provide dosages, and deal with your particular situation.

TABLE OF CONTENTS

IVERMECTIN

Ivermectin is a drug that has been the subject of much debate and interest lately because of its potential use in the treatment of a number of illnesses, most notably parasitic infections and, more significantly, the COVID-19 pandemic. This is a revised description of ivermectin:

Ivermectin: What is it?

The drug ivermectin was first created in the 1970s and is made from a substance that is present in Streptomyces avermitilis, a particular kind of bacteria. It is a member of the antiparasitic agent drug class. For many years, ivermectin has been used to treat a variety of parasite illnesses in both humans and animals.

What Ivermectin Does Not Do?

Ivermectin acts by impairing the parasites' ability to use their muscles and nerves, which causes paralysis and ultimately death. It accomplishes this by attaching itself to specific neurotransmitters that are necessary for these organisms to operate normally, most notably gamma-aminobutyric acid (GABA). Because this impairment of neurotransmitter action is unique to parasites, at standard therapeutic levels it has no negative effects on humans or most other animals.

Usage of Ivermectin Commonly:

Ivermectin is mainly used to treat a variety of parasitic infections, such as the following:

Onchocerciasis, or river blindness
Encephalitis lymphatica
Scabies
Strongyloidiasis in the stomach
Both pubic and head lice (pediculosis).
Veterinary Health Care: In veterinary medicine, ivermectin is frequently used to prevent and cure parasite diseases in pets and animals.

Disputes Regarding Ivermectin:

Ivermectin attracted a lot of interest as a possible COVID-19 treatment during the pandemic. According to certain research, it may possess antiviral capabilities against SARS-CoV-2, the virus that causes COVID-19.

Ivermectin therapy for COVID-19, however, is still very debatable and the topic of constant research and discussion. Health authorities and medical professionals had not approved it as a regular treatment or endorsed its routine usage for COVID-19 as of September 2021, when I last updated my information.

Crucial Points to Remember:

Only a licensed healthcare provider's advice and prescription should be followed when taking ivermectin.
The particular ailment being treated determines the dosage and length of treatment.
When taken as directed, ivermectin is usually well accepted; but, as with any medicine, there may be side effects

that need to be discussed with a healthcare professional.

Please be aware that after my last knowledge update, the situation with ivermectin may have changed. For the most up-to-date information on its usage, possible advantages, and hazards, it's vital to consult the most recent research and medical guidelines. Always seek the guidance of a medical practitioner for specific medical advice.

ALTERNATIVE TREATMENTS

Therapeutic modalities that are employed in addition to or instead of traditional medical treatments are referred to as alternative treatments. These alternative therapies might include a broad spectrum of interventions and therapies, frequently emphasizing natural remedies and holistic well-being. It's crucial to remember that there can be large variations in the safety and efficacy of alternative therapies. As such, people should always seek the advice of medical specialists before pursuing alternative therapies, particularly for serious medical illnesses. The following alternative therapies are listed along with a thorough description of each:

acupuncture

The ancient Chinese art of acupuncture involves the insertion of tiny needles into predetermined body sites. Its foundation is the idea of achieving equilibrium with the body's life force, or "qi."

Uses: Acupuncture is frequently used to treat a range of chronic diseases as well as pain, tension, and anxiety.

Herbal Remedies:

Description: Herbal medicine treats and prevents health problems by using plants, herbs, and botanicals. These cures can be found in a variety of forms, including tinctures, teas, and supplements.

Applications: Herbal medicine is used to treat a variety of ailments, such as digestion issues, pain management, and immune system support.

Homoeopathy

Homeopathy operates under the principle that "like cures like." It uses extremely diluted chemicals with the idea of promoting the body's own healing mechanisms.

Uses: Although its efficacy is debatable, homeopathy is frequently used to treat allergies, colds, and other acute ailments.

Chiropractic Treatment:

The diagnosis and treatment of musculoskeletal diseases, especially those pertaining to the spine, are the main goals of chiropractic care. It requires manual modifications and changes.

Applications: Chiropractors frequently treat headaches, neck and back discomfort.

Aromatherapy:

Description: Aromatherapy is the use of plant-derived essential oils to enhance mental, emotional, and physical health. You can massage with these oils, apply them topically, or inhale them.

Applications: Aromatherapy is frequently used to promote mood, reduce tension, and promote relaxation.

Chinese traditional medicine (TCM):

TCM is a comprehensive medical approach that uses nutritional therapy, herbal remedies, acupuncture, and physical therapies like Tai Chi. Its foundation is the Yin and Yang, or life energy, balance of the body.

Applications: Traditional Chinese medicine (TCM) treats a variety of ailments, such as gynecological problems, digestive problems, and chronic pain.

Naturopathy:

Naturopathy is the study of natural medicine, which includes herbal remedies, dietary modifications, lifestyle adjustments, and other natural therapies. It seeks to address the underlying causes of disease.

Applications: Naturopathic doctors treat a range of illnesses, from chronic illnesses to allergies.

Mindfulness & Meditation:

These approaches, which include deep breathing and meditation, are meant to train the mind to attain mental clarity, emotional stability, and stress reduction.

Applications: Mindfulness and meditation are used to enhance general mental health and manage stress, anxiety, and depression.

Yoga:

Yoga is a physical, mental, and spiritual discipline that enhances mental and physical health through postures, breathing techniques, and meditation.

Applications: Yoga is well known for enhancing strength, flexibility, and lowering stress.

Massage Therapy:

Massage therapy is a therapeutic approach that aims to relieve muscle tension, enhance circulation, and foster relaxation by manipulating the body's soft tissues.

Uses: Reducing stress, managing pain, and enhancing general physical well-being are among its frequent uses. When considering alternative therapies, care must be taken, particularly for severe or long-term medical disorders. Always seek the advice of a licensed healthcare provider to be sure that these treatments are suitable and safe for your particular medical needs. The goal of integrative medicine is to offer a more thorough and individualized healthcare experience by combining traditional and alternative treatments.

RESILIENCE AND DURABILITY

In the context of healthcare, resistance and sustainability mostly refer to two different but related concepts:

1. Opposition to Drugs or Therapies:

The development of resistance in microorganisms, such as viruses, bacteria, or parasites, is the result of their ability to resist the effects of drugs or treatments that were once effective against them. This may make treatments that were once successful useless.

Causes: Genetic alterations in the bacteria or usage or abuse of treatments, like antibiotics or antiparasitic therapies, can lead to resistance. Resilient microorganisms are able to endure and procreate, transferring their resistance to new generations.

Consequences: Treatment failure, greater rates of morbidity and death, longer hospital stays, and increased healthcare expenses can all result from drug resistance. It is a problem for public health worldwide.

2. Healthcare Sustainability:

The practice of providing medical care and conducting research in a way that reduces environmental effect, conserves resources, and guarantees that healthcare systems can satisfy the requirements of present and future generations is known as sustainability in the healthcare industry.

Aspects: There are various facets of healthcare sustainability, such as:

Environmental Sustainability: Cutting waste, adopting eco-friendly procedures, and minimizing the carbon impact of healthcare institutions.

Economic sustainability refers to preventing resource misuse, keeping healthcare expenses under control, and ensuring that healthcare systems are both profitable and efficient.

Social Sustainability: Encouraging health education and prevention, resolving gaps, and granting equal access to healthcare services.

Benefits: Using sustainable healthcare practices can save money, protect the environment, enhance public health, and create a more robust healthcare system.

The junction between sustainability and resistance:

The viability of healthcare systems might be jeopardized by resistance to drugs and therapies. Drug-resistant illnesses have the potential to increase healthcare expenses, lengthen hospital stays, and necessitate more resource-intensive treatments as they grow more common.

Sustainable healthcare practices can slow down the emergence of drug resistance. One such practice is the prudent use of antibiotics. Antibiotic stewardship initiatives, for instance, seek to minimize antibiotic use in order to lower resistance.

On the other hand, by retaining the efficacy of current treatments and lowering the need for expensive alternatives, treating drug resistance can support the sustainability of healthcare.

In summary, sustainability in healthcare relates to the conscientious use of resources, the influence on the environment, and fair access to care, whereas resistance in healthcare refers to the capacity of germs to withstand the effects of medications. These two ideas overlap in that treating resistance can guarantee that treatments continue to be successful and efficient, which helps support the long-term viability of healthcare systems. On the other hand, drug resistance can be stopped from developing and spreading with the support of sustainable healthcare practices.

IMPACT ON GLOBAL HEALTH

The term "global health impact" describes the extensive effects, both favorable and unfavorable, of health-related problems, treatments, and regulations on a worldwide level. It covers a wide range of variables, including population health and the political, social, and economic effects of health-related actions. This is a thorough description of how it affects world health:

1. State of Health and Well-Being:

Benefits: Longer life expectancy, lower morbidity, and more general well-being are all brought about by improved global health. This progress is attributed to advancements in healthcare, immunization programs, and disease prevention activities.

Negative Impact: There can be major health inequities that impede well-being due to health disparities and the burden of diseases like HIV/AIDS, malaria, and non-communicable diseases.

2. Economic Effect:

Positive Impact: Productivity increases and economic growth can be facilitated by a healthy population. Economic development can be boosted by lower healthcare costs, higher labor force participation, and better education brought about by improved health.

Negative Effects: Health emergencies, such pandemics or epidemics, can cause large financial losses due to medical costs, lost production, and hiccups in trade and tourism.

3. Systems of Healthcare:

Positive Impact: By enhancing infrastructure, staff training, and access to necessary medical services, global health efforts help fortify healthcare systems. This improves a nation's ability to address health-related issues. Negative effects include insufficient care, a lack of resources, and restricted access to healthcare services as a result of weak healthcare systems' inability to meet the demands of their respective populations.

4. Control and Prevention of Diseases:

Positive Impact: Vaccination campaigns and attempts to combat neglected tropical illnesses, among other global efforts to prevent and control diseases, have saved countless lives and lessened suffering.

Negative effects include extensive illness, death, and disruption of society when infectious disease control efforts fail to contain epidemics and pandemics.

5. Effect on the Environment:

Positive Impact: Climate change-related health risks are decreased and environmental preservation is aided by sustainable health practices, such as lowering carbon emissions from transportation and healthcare facilities.

Negative Effect: Ecosystems and public health can be adversely impacted by poor health practices, such as the incorrect disposal of medical waste or the use of pharmaceuticals that are detrimental to the environment.

6. Impact on Society and Politics:

Positive Impact: Through programs like the Sustainable Development Goals (SDGs) and organizations like the World Health Organization (WHO), improved global health can foster social stability, lessen conflict, and increase international collaboration.

Negative Effect: Health crises can worsen already-existing inequities, put pressure on political systems, and cause social unrest. Healthcare access has the potential to become a divisive political issue.

7. Human rights and health equity:

Positive Impact: Addressing health inequities and advancing human rights are common components of efforts to enhance global health. The protection of disadvantaged populations and fair access to healthcare are the goals of these programs.

Negative effects include discrimination, human rights breaches, and systemic injustices stemming from inadequate access to healthcare.

8. Innovation and Research:

Positive Impact: Innovation and research in global health promote medical progress, resulting in novel therapies, diagnostic instruments, and technology that help people all over the world.

Negative Effect: Research and innovation funding shortages can impede the development of novel therapies and interventions and impede efforts to solve global health concerns.

To sum up, the term "global health impact" refers to the extensive effects of health-related variables on a worldwide level. Health inequities, environmental degradation, and social and political instability all have negative effects, whereas economic growth, enhanced healthcare systems, and better well-being can have positive effects. International cooperation, infrastructure investments in the healthcare sector, and a dedication to human rights and health equity are all necessary to address the difficulties facing global health.

ADMINISTRATION & DOSAGE

Information about dosage and administration is essential to healthcare and drug use. To guarantee the efficacy and safety of pharmaceuticals and medical treatments, it offers instructions on how to correctly prescribe, administer, and take them. This is a thorough description of administration and dosage:

1. Dosage

Definition: Dosage is the quantity of a drug or treatment that a doctor prescribes or suggests a patient take in order to get the intended therapeutic result.

Variables Affecting Dosage:

Patient's Weight and Age: A patient's weight, age, and developmental stage can all affect the dosage.
Condition Severity: The dosage may vary depending on how serious the ailment is that needs to be treated.
Route of Administration: Various dosages may be needed for oral, injectable, topical, and other routes of administration.
Patient's Health Status: The dosage may be impacted by the patient's general health, particularly liver and renal function.
Drug Interactions: When deciding on a dosage, it is important to take into account any possible interactions with other medications a patient may be taking.

Different dose forms such as pills, capsules, liquid solutions, injections, creams, and more are available for medications. The recommended dose may change depending on the dosage type used.

Dose Frequency: The frequency of dosing (e.g., once daily, twice daily, every four hours) for a medicine is also specified in the dosage instructions.

Loading dosage: To quickly reach therapeutic levels in the body, a loading dosage, which is a higher initial dose, may occasionally be administered. This is followed by a lower maintenance dose.

2. Management:

Definition: The procedure of giving a patient a medication or other therapy is referred to as administration.

Administrative Paths:

Oral: The digestive tract is used to consume and absorb medications administered orally.
Intravenous (IV): Drugs are injected via a vein straight into the bloodstream.
Intramuscular (IM): A muscle is injected with medication so that it can be absorbed.
Subcutaneous (SC or SQ): Medications are injected into fatty tissue, usually just beneath the skin.
Topical: Drugs are absorbed through the skin after being applied to the skin's surface.

Inhalation: Nebulizers or inhalers are devices that provide medication straight to the respiratory system.

Rectal: The rectum is used to give medication.

Intrathecal: The spinal canal is used to provide medication.

Correct Technique: To guarantee that the medication reaches its target location and is absorbed appropriately, accurate and exact administration techniques are essential.

Use of Devices: Certain tools, such inhalers, syringes, or infusion pumps, could be needed for administration. When using these devices, patients and healthcare providers need to be properly trained.

Adherence: To guarantee the medication's efficacy, patients must carefully follow the directions for administration.

3. Education of Patients:

To make sure that patients understand how to take their medications or receive treatments correctly, patient education is essential. This includes describing the dosage, the method of administration, the time, and any special directions (such taking it with or without meals).

4. Safety Points to Remember:

To avoid mistakes, pharmaceutical safety involves making sure the right drug, dose, and delivery method are used.

Precise dosage and monitoring are necessary for medications with a narrow therapeutic index in order to prevent side effects or insufficient therapy.

5. Measurement

Titration, which begins with a low dose and increases it gradually until the intended therapeutic benefit is reached or the side effects become unacceptable, is required for certain drugs.

6. Considering Children and the Elderly:

Because adolescent and geriatric individuals differ in their metabolism, organ function, and tolerance, different dosing and administration protocols may apply.

7. Customization:

Depending on the particular traits and medical background of each patient, healthcare professionals frequently customize dosage and administration.

8. Observation and Modifications:

As needed, dose or administration changes may result from ongoing patient monitoring in order to preserve the intended therapeutic impact and reduce adverse effects.

9. Record-keeping:

Maintaining accurate records is crucial for monitoring the administration of medications, patient reactions, and any negative consequences.

To sum up, following dosage and administration guidelines is essential to the safe and efficient use of prescription drugs and medical procedures. They need accuracy and focus from both patients and healthcare practitioners, and they take into consideration a variety of patient-specific aspects. In order to minimize the risk of side effects and achieve the desired treatment outcomes, proper education and adherence are crucial.

INSTRUCTION FOR PATIENTS

Patient education is a vital aspect of healthcare that gives people the power to decide for themselves what is best for their health and wellbeing. It includes giving patients the knowledge, tools, and support they need to comprehend their medical issues, available treatments, and successful health management techniques. This is a thorough description of patient education:

1. Patient Education Is Vital

Making Informed Decisions: Patient education guarantees that people possess the information and comprehension required to actively engage in healthcare decision-making.

This entails selecting therapies, prescription drugs, and lifestyle modifications with knowledge.

Disease Prevention: Informing patients about screening, immunization, and healthy lifestyle choices can help lower their chance of contracting an illness or having it worsen.

Treatment Adherence: Patients with better health outcomes are more likely to follow their recommended drugs and therapies if they are aware of their treatment plans.

Self-Management: Patient education gives people the knowledge and self-assurance they need to take care of chronic illnesses, keep an eye on their symptoms, and know when to contact a doctor.

Better Communication: Knowledgeable patients are better equipped to ask insightful questions and offer insightful comments to improve the standard of care while speaking with healthcare professionals.

2. Essential Elements of Patient Instruction:

Information sharing: Giving patients pertinent, precise, and understandable information about their diagnosis, course of treatment, and prognosis.

Ensuring that patients receive information in a comprehensible manner, irrespective of their literacy proficiency or background, is known as health literacy.

Encouraging direct and honest communication between patients and medical professionals so that the former can voice concerns and ask questions.

Interactive learning involves including patients in conversations, exercises, and practical learning experiences to strengthen comprehension.

Multimodal Approaches: To accommodate diverse learning styles, a range of instructional resources, including written materials, films, diagrams, and digital tools, are used.

3. Patient Education Procedure:

Assessment: Medical professionals determine the patient's level of understanding, requirements, and treatment choices.

Planning: Based on the patient's assessment, a customized educational plan is created, taking into consideration their objectives and unique situation.

Implementation: One-on-one conversations, group meetings, instructional materials, or internet resources are used to provide patient education.

Reinforcement: In order to expand and preserve their knowledge of health, patients are urged to routinely examine and use the information.

Evaluation: To make sure patients are making educated decisions and properly managing their health, the efficacy of the education is evaluated by surveys, follow-up conversations, and clinical results.

4. Subjects Included in Patient Instruction:

Understanding the nature of the medical illness, how it progresses, and its possible outcomes is known as diagnosis and prognosis.

Treatment Options: Outlining the advantages, disadvantages, and side effects of the various treatments.

Teaching patients about recommended drugs, dosages, schedules, and any interactions is known as medication management.

Lifestyle modification: giving advice on nutrition, physical activity, quitting smoking, handling stress, and other aspects of daily living that can affect one's health.

Self-Monitoring: Assisting patients in keeping a record of their symptoms, vital signs, or other medical information.

Promoting immunizations, screenings, and routine check-ups are examples of preventive measures.

Safety Measures: Giving patients advice on how to handle crises and unfavorable situations.

5. Obstacles in Patient Instruction:

Health Literacy: Ensuring that patients with different degrees of health literacy can access and comprehend information.

Understanding and honoring cultural variations and beliefs that could influence medical decisions is known as cultural sensitivity.

Language Barriers: Overcoming language obstacles for patients who don't speak the healthcare provider's native tongue.

Time Restrictions: During appointments, healthcare providers might not have enough time to give thorough instruction.

Healthcare Disparities: Resolving differences in how various people are able to access resources for healthcare and education.

6. Technology and Instruction for Patients:

Patient education is being delivered remotely more frequently thanks to the use of digital tools and telehealth platforms, which increase accessibility and convenience.

Patients can always access instructional materials and support through mobile apps, internet resources, and virtual support groups.

7. Empowerment of Patients:

By enabling people to actively participate in their healthcare, patient education improves quality of life and results in better health outcomes.

Patients who feel empowered are more likely to follow their treatment regimens and take preventative actions.

In conclusion, patient education is a critical component of healthcare that enables people to effectively manage their health, make educated decisions, and take an active role in their own treatment. In the end, it leads to better health outcomes and a higher quality of life by fostering enhanced communication between patients and healthcare professionals and improving health literacy.

CLINICAL INVESTIGATIONS

Clinical trials are investigations aimed at assessing the efficacy, safety, and possible advantages or disadvantages of medications, medical devices, therapies, interventions, or healthcare tactics in human participants. These trials are critical to the advancement of medical knowledge, the creation of novel therapeutics, the enhancement of current treatments, and the security of healthcare interventions. A thorough description of clinical trials can be found here:

1. Why Conduct Clinical Trials?

Efficacy and Safety: Clinical trials seek to evaluate the safety of a medical intervention as well as its efficacy in treating or preventing a particular medical disease. Examples of these interventions include drugs, vaccines, and surgical procedures.

Comparative Studies: To determine which treatment or intervention is more effective or has fewer negative effects, several clinical trials evaluate various approaches or therapies.

Disease preventive: Vaccines and lifestyle modifications are two examples of disease preventive tactics that may be the subject of clinical trials.

Diagnostic Tests: Clinical trials can assess the precision and usefulness of imaging methods or diagnostic tests.

Quality of Life: Certain studies investigate how treatments affect patients' physical, mental, and social well-being as well as their overall quality of life.

2. Clinical Trial Phases:

Phase I: These studies evaluate the intervention's dose and safety in small groups of healthy participants.

Phase II: Phase II trials evaluate the safety, effectiveness, and side effects of the intervention on a broader set of patients. Researchers explore for early indications of efficacy.

Phase III: A bigger patient group is participating in Phase III studies, which are designed to monitor side effects, establish the effectiveness of the intervention, and compare it with standard therapies or placebos.

Phase IV: Often referred to as post-marketing trials, Phase IV research takes place following a treatment's approval and widespread distribution. They keep an eye on long-term efficacy, safety, and any uncommon adverse events in a bigger patient base.

3. Research Framework:

Randomized Controlled Trials (RCTs): In these studies, participants are assigned at random to one of two groups: the treatment group, which receives the intervention, and the control group, which receives a placebo or standard treatment. The gold standard of clinical research is regarded as being RCTs.

Studies employing observational methods: In observational methods, subjects are observed and data are gathered from them without any intervention. These studies are frequently used to evaluate treatment outcomes, natural history of diseases, and risk factors.

Cross-Over Trials: These trials allow comparisons within the same subjects by enabling participants who were initially allocated to one group to switch to the other group after a certain amount of time.

4. Knowledgeable Consent:

Clinical study participation is voluntary, and participants must give their informed consent. This indicates that before consenting to participate, participants were fully informed about the goals, risks, rewards, and options of the study.

5. Research Subjects:

Clinical trial participants may comprise persons with particular medical disorders, specified groups, or healthy volunteers, contingent upon the goals of the research.

6. Ethical Points to Remember:

To guarantee participant safety and the study's scientific validity, clinical trials must abide by ethical norms such as informed consent, patient confidentiality, and oversight by

Institutional Review Boards (IRBs) or Ethics Committees.

7. Gathering and Examining Data:

Throughout the experiment, data is gathered to evaluate efficacy and safety. To ascertain the effectiveness of the intervention and the statistical significance of any detected differences, statistical analysis is employed.

8. Publication and Reporting:

To share findings with the scientific and medical communities, trial results are usually published in medical publications. Reporting is essential to peer review and transparency.

9. Approval by Regulation:

Regulatory bodies (like the FDA and EMA) must approve new medications, vaccines, medical devices, or treatments for general use once they have undergone successful clinical trials.

10. Advantages and Dangers:

Enrolling in a clinical trial may provide advantages including getting access to state-of-the-art therapies. But there are also possible risks associated with it, such as the possibility of experiencing a placebo or unidentified adverse effects.

11. Clinical Trials' Importance

The foundation of evidence-based medicine is clinical trials, which give medical decision-makers a scientific foundation while also enhancing patient care.

To sum up, clinical trials are critical to improving patient safety, assessing medicines, and expanding medical knowledge. They employ a strict procedure to evaluate the safety and effectiveness of medical interventions, which eventually improves patient care and healthcare outcomes.

COLCHICINE WITH IVERMECTIN

The antiparasitic medication ivermectin has drawn debate and attention in relation to COVID-19. It's crucial to note that major health agencies, such as the World Health Organization (WHO) and the U.S. Food and Drug Administration (FDA), had not universally acknowledged the use of ivermectin as a conventional treatment for COVID-19 as of my last knowledge update in September 2021. Yet, investigations and conversations about its possible application in the prevention and treatment of COVID-19 were still underway. This is a thorough explanation of ivermectin's connection to COVID-19:

1. Overview of Ivermectin:

The main purpose of the FDA-approved medication ivermectin is to treat parasite infections in both people and animals. It works well on a variety of parasites, including as mites, intestinal worms, and some ectoparasites.

2. Initial Interest in COVID-19 Ivermectin:

Early laboratory research on the COVID-19 pandemic revealed that ivermectin may possess antiviral qualities and be able to prevent the SARS-CoV-2 virus from replicating in cell cultures.

Ivermectin's potential as a COVID-19 treatment has drawn interest as a result of these first findings.

3. Clinical Research and Debate:

Ivermectin's potential for use in COVID-19 treatment and prevention has been the subject of numerous clinical trials and observational research.

Positive results with ivermectin treatment for COVID-19 patients included decreased viral loads, faster recovery periods, and decreased death rates, according to certain research.

Nevertheless, several of these studies had drawbacks, including inconsistent findings, limited sample sizes, and methodological errors.

4. Conflicting Evidence

Major health agencies like the FDA, WHO, and National Institutes of Health (NIH) had not recommended the normal use of ivermectin for COVID-19 outside of research studies as of my last update in September 2021.

It was thought that there was insufficient data to form firm conclusions about the effectiveness of ivermectin in treating COVID-19. Therefore, additional high-quality randomized controlled trials were required.

5. Safety Issues:

Particularly when taken in larger dosages, ivermectin can have adverse effects such as nausea, vomiting, diarrhea, and, in rare instances, more serious reactions such liver damage and neurologic problems.

When ivermectin formulations meant for animals are misused, harmful effects can occur in humans.

6. Regulatory Measures:

Ivermectin for COVID-19 has been approved for usage in some nations and areas under specific conditions, while its use has been restricted in others or is advised against.

Regulatory bodies have cautioned against using ivermectin formulations derived from animals improperly to treat COVID-19 in people.

7. Current Research:

More clinical trials and systematic reviews are being carried out as part of the ongoing investigation into the possible advantages and disadvantages of ivermectin for COVID-19.

8. Professional Views:

The lack of agreement regarding the role of ivermectin in COVID-19 highlights the significance of seeking advice from credible health organizations and speaking with medical experts when making specific medical decisions.

Regarding the use of ivermectin for COVID-19, it's critical to stay current with the most recent research and advice from health authorities, as the situation and guidelines may have changed since my September 2021 update. The general consensus at the time was that additional solid clinical data was required to decide whether ivermectin should be used as a first line of treatment for COVID-19.

METHOD OF ACTION

The precise biological or biochemical processes that a medication, therapeutic agent, or treatment uses to influence the body are referred to as the mechanism of action (MoA). In order to create and use medicines in a safe and effective manner, pharmaceutical companies, researchers, and healthcare professionals must have a thorough understanding of the MoA. This is a thorough description of the action's mechanism:

1. Attachment to Specific Molecules:

The majority of medications and therapeutic substances function by interacting with particular molecules or bodily targets. These targets may consist of nucleic acids, proteins, enzymes, receptors, or other parts of the cell.

The medication has a very particular binding affinity. Hydrogen bonds, electrostatic contacts, and hydrophobic interactions are a few of the forces that might cause this interaction.

2. Modified Molecular Operations:

The medication has the ability to change a target molecule's activity or function once it has bound to it. This can happen via a number of mechanisms:

Enzyme Inhibition: Certain medications hinder the ability of enzymes to perform their regular metabolic reactions by inhibiting their activity. Statins, for instance, block the enzyme HMG-CoA reductase, which is necessary for the manufacture of cholesterol.

Receptor Modulation: Substances can alter cell signaling pathways by activating or blocking particular cell surface receptors. For example, beta-blockers lower heart rate by blocking beta-adrenergic receptors in the heart.

Ion Channel Modulation: Ion channels in cell membranes regulate the flow of ions such as calcium, potassium, and sodium. Some medications alter these channels. Both muscle contraction and nerve conduction may be impacted by this.

Drugs used in cancer treatment, in particular, have the ability to bind to DNA and alter its structure or function, which stops cells from proliferating.

3. Impact of Pharmacology:

Certain pharmacological effects result from the drug's target molecule's altered function. These outcomes may be beneficial (desired) or harmful (undesired).

Depending on the drug's intended use, therapeutic benefits could include decreased inflammation, lowering blood pressure, pain alleviation, or prevention of microbiological development.

4. Physiological and Cellular Reactions:

The body experiences cellular and physiological reactions as a result of the drug's pharmacological effects at the molecular level.

An example of a pain reliever that reduces inflammation and pain at the site of injury is ibuprofen, which inhibits an enzyme involved in the manufacture of prostaglandins.

5. Effects: Local versus Systemic:

The drug's characteristics and mode of administration determine whether the MoA will have systemic or local effects.

Topical creams used to treat skin diseases are examples of products with localized effects.

When a medication enters the bloodstream and impacts distant tissues or organs, this is known as a systemic effect. When taking oral drugs or receiving intravenous injections, this is typical.

6. Dosage-Response Association:

The pharmacological dosage and the MoA are frequently associated. Although higher doses may have more noticeable effects, there is a greater chance that they will cause negative side effects.

The dose-response relationship aids in figuring out the best dosage to maximize therapeutic benefits and reduce adverse effects.

7. Timeline of Operations:

The molecular weight of a medicine determines its duration, onset, and peak of activity. Certain medications take effect quickly and give relief right away, while others take longer to take effect but have more potent benefits.

It is essential to comprehend the time course when it comes to dosing and patient care.

8. Resistance and Tolerance:

Chronic drug use might cause the body to become less receptive to the effects of the drug due to adaptation (tolerance). Furthermore, bacteria can become resistant to antibiotics.

This calls for changing the dosage of medications or utilizing different therapies.

9. Adverse Reactions and Effects:

Comprehending the moA aids in anticipating possible drug interactions and adverse consequences. Certain medications may contend for the same target molecules, which could result in unfavorable responses or interactions.

To sum up, a drug's mechanism of action provides a thorough description of how it interacts with particular molecules in the body to achieve its pharmacological or therapeutic effects. It involves chemical binding, changes in how molecules function, as well as cellular and physiological reactions. It may have both positive therapeutic effects and unfavorable side effects. For the creation of safe and efficient drugs as well as for clinical usage, a thorough understanding of the MoA is necessary.

SAFETY AND ADVERSE REACTIONS

Safety and side effects are important considerations in medicine and healthcare. They deal with the possible dangers, side effects, and safety measures related to medical treatments, such as medications, devices, and therapies. Healthcare professionals and patients alike must comprehend side effects and guarantee safety. The following provides a thorough discussion of side effects, safety precautions, and their importance:

1. Inverse Effects:

Definition: Side effects are unexpected and frequently undesirable outcomes that come from using a pharmaceutical, medical device, or healthcare intervention. They are sometimes referred to as unwanted effects or unfavorable reactions.

Kinds of Adverse Effects:

Common Side Effects: These are often modest side effects that many people taking a specific medicine encounter on a regular basis. Headache, nausea, and drowsiness are a few examples.

Serious Side Effects: Though less often, these can be extremely dangerous or even fatal. An important drop in blood pressure, allergic responses, and organ damage are a few examples.

Onset: Adverse effects may start as soon as a medication is taken (acute side effects) or may appear gradually over time with continued use (chronic side effects).

Certain adverse effects are dose-dependent, meaning that increasing a drug's dosage will make them worse.

2. Safety Points to Remember:

Safety Profile: A medication's or medical intervention safety profile is a thorough evaluation of all possible adverse effects, drug interactions, contraindications, and general safety in different patient populations.

Risk-Benefit Assessment: Patients and medical professionals need to balance the possible advantages of a treatment with any associated hazards. An alternate course of treatment may be considered in certain situations, while in others the advantages of the treatment may exceed the hazards.

Special Populations: People who belong to specialized populations, such the elderly, youngsters, or pregnant women, may be more susceptible to certain side effects or need special safety measures.

3. Observation and Documentation:

Monitoring: Throughout therapy, patients and medical professionals should keep an eye out for any adverse effects. It could be required to have routine examinations and monitoring in order to quickly identify and treat harmful responses.

Reporting: In order to support the continuous evaluation of pharmaceutical safety, healthcare practitioners are urged to report adverse occurrences to regulatory bodies, such as the FDA's MedWatch program in the United States.

4. Patient information and labeling:

Essential safety information is provided through patient information inserts and comprehensive labeling on medications and medical equipment. This covers cautions, possible adverse effects, dosage guidelines, and contraindications.

5. Informed Consent and Communication:

It is critical that patients and healthcare professionals communicate in an honest and open manner. All treatments should come with a complete disclosure to patients regarding any possible adverse effects and safety concerns.

Legal and ethical requirements for informed consent guarantee that patients are aware of the advantages and disadvantages of a treatment before consenting to it.

6. Vigilance with drugs:

The research and practices around the identification, evaluation, comprehension, and avoidance of side effects or any other medication-related issues are known as pharmacovigilance.

Pharmacies and regulatory bodies keep a close eye on the safety of pharmaceuticals and may respond by issuing recalls or warnings in response to new safety issues.

7. Techniques for Mitigating Risk:

To reduce possible harm, several drugs and procedures call for particular risk mitigation techniques. This can involve restricted distribution, patient education, or testing that is required.

8. Regulatory Authorization:

Regulatory bodies thoroughly test a drug or medical device in preclinical and clinical studies to determine its safety profile before approving it for use. Permission is given when advantages exceed disadvantages.

9. Juggling Safety and Effectiveness:

Healthcare professionals must carefully strike a balance between the necessity of ensuring patient safety and the requirement to deliver effective therapies. This entails deciding which therapy alternatives are best for each patient based on their unique traits and medical background.

To sum up, safety and side effects are important factors to take into account while making healthcare decisions. Ensuring safe and effective healthcare interventions requires patients and healthcare practitioners to communicate openly, monitor for adverse events, and understand the potential risks and benefits of treatments. The safety profiles of pharmaceuticals and medical devices are continuously improved because of ongoing research and regulatory control.

ACCEPTED APPLICATIONS

The term "approved uses" describes the particular illnesses, ailments, or indications for which a medication, medical device, or therapeutic intervention has received formal approval from regulatory bodies like the European Medicines Agency (EMA) in the European Union or the U.S. Food and Drug Administration (FDA) in the United States. The product's approval signifies that it has passed stringent testing and been shown to be both safe and effective in treating or managing specific medical problems. Here is a thorough breakdown of permitted uses:

1. Regulatory Authorization:

Drugs and medical devices must be evaluated and approved by regulatory bodies before being marketed or used within their respective jurisdictions. Examples of these agencies are the FDA in the United States, the EMA in the European Union, Health Canada, and others globally.

A thorough examination of preclinical and clinical data provided by pharmaceutical or medical device companies is a necessary step in the approval process.

2. Medical Trials:

Manufacturers are required to carry out comprehensive clinical research to prove the product's safety and effectiveness before applying for approval.

Preclinical research, Phase I (safety), Phase II (efficacy), and Phase III (large-scale efficacy and safety trials) are the standard phases of clinical trials.

3. Significance of Approval:

Known as "indications," approved uses are particular medical problems or diseases for which a medication or medical device has been shown to be both safe and effective.

All authorized indications are documented in the official product documentation or labeling and backed by evidence from clinical trials.

4. Product Information and Labeling:

Manufacturers are required by regulatory bodies to include comprehensive information about the allowed uses of their products in product labeling, packaging inserts, and other official documentation.

Healthcare practitioners can better comprehend the conditions under which the product is prescribed or used with the use of this information.

5. Off-Label Utilization:

Sometimes medical professionals will use medications or devices outside of their permitted indications. We refer to this as "off-label use."

Off-label usage is often based on clinical judgment and evidence, and it may contain hazards, even if it is legal and may be clinically appropriate in some circumstances.

6. Orphan and Pediatric Indications:

Based on pediatric clinical trials, several medications are approved specifically for use in pediatric populations, ensuring that children receive safe and effective care.

For the treatment of uncommon diseases, orphan drug designations and approvals are given, which encourages the development of remedies that might not be commercially feasible without such support.

7. Extension of Significance:

Manufacturers may apply for clearance for additional indications beyond the ones for which they were first approved if further data becomes available.

A medication's indications may be expanded to enable use for more medical disorders or in a wider range of patient demographics.

8. After-the-Market Monitoring

Regulatory bodies use post-market monitoring to keep an eye on the efficacy and safety of medications and medical devices even after they have been approved.

Regulatory bodies have the authority to change approved indications, add warnings, or even revoke permission in the event of safety issues or unfavorable events.

9. Relevance of Permitted Uses:

Healthcare practitioners can prescribe or utilize medications and medical devices safely and effectively with the help of approved uses, which offer a clear framework.

Based on thorough scientific analysis, they assist in ensuring that patients receive the right treatments for their unique medical situations.

To sum up, approved uses are the particular medical ailments or illnesses that a medication, medical gadget, or treatment intervention has been officially approved by regulatory bodies to treat. These approvals are crucial for assisting medical practitioners in prescribing or utilizing these medications correctly and safely to improve patient health because they are founded on a thorough examination of clinical trial data.

Made in the USA
Monee, IL
23 July 2025

21743061R00056